My Mommy is a Nurse.

She tells me about her days at work.

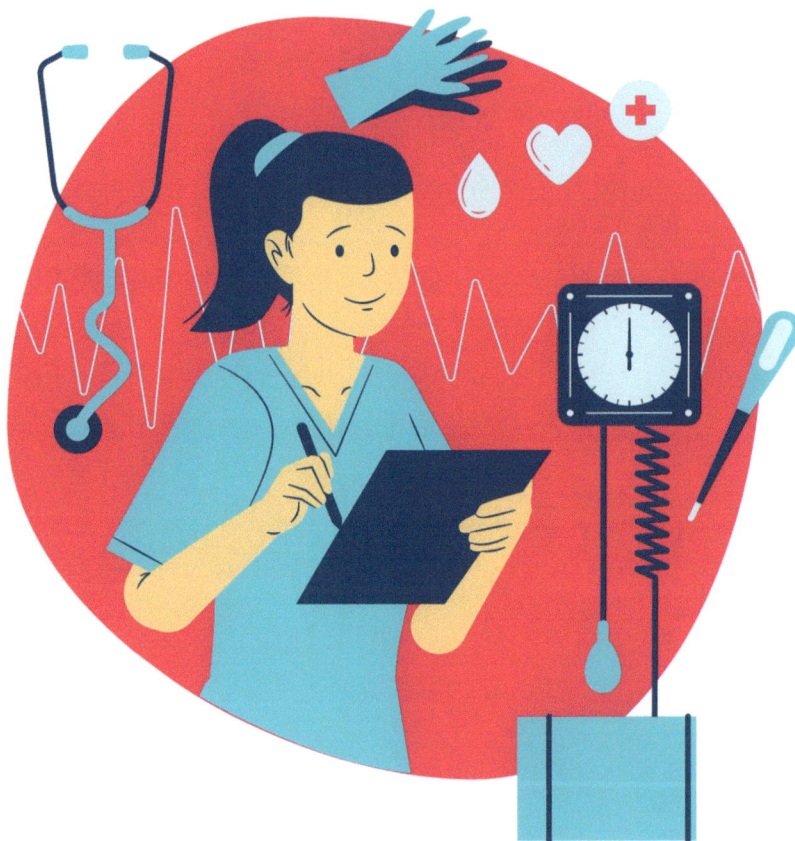

She says "There are good days and bad days."

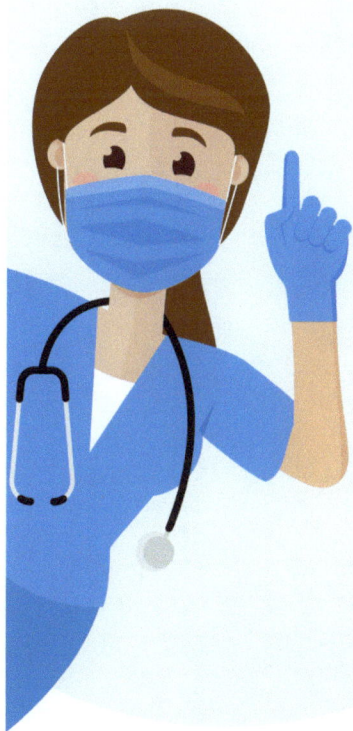

It's okay to have BAD DAYS

I have learned that nurses do many things.

Here are some things that my Mom
does as a nurse.

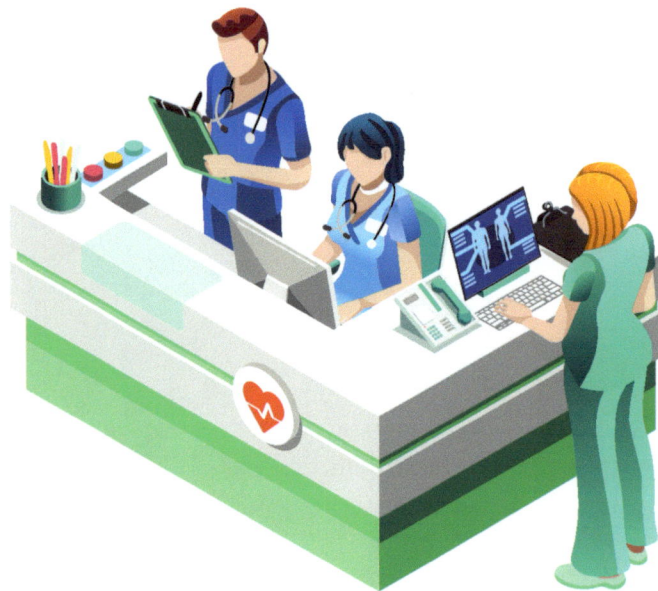

She gives her patients medications only after making sure it is safe to do so.

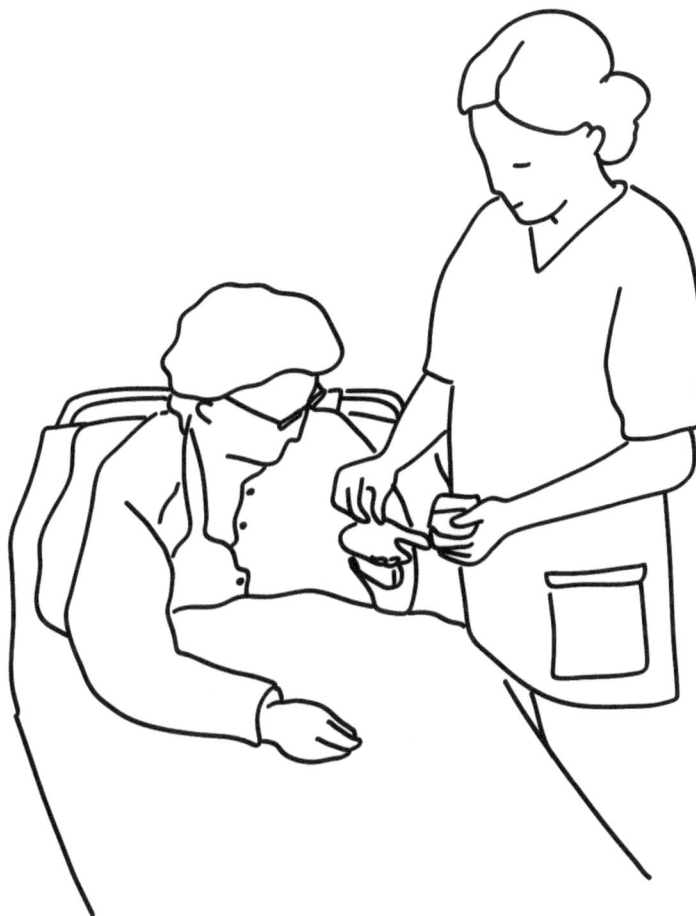

She tells me this is called the five rights.

Right Patient
Right Time
Right Dose
Right Route
Right Medicine

Each of her patients gets an assessment. She examines them from head to toe and asks them questions about their body.

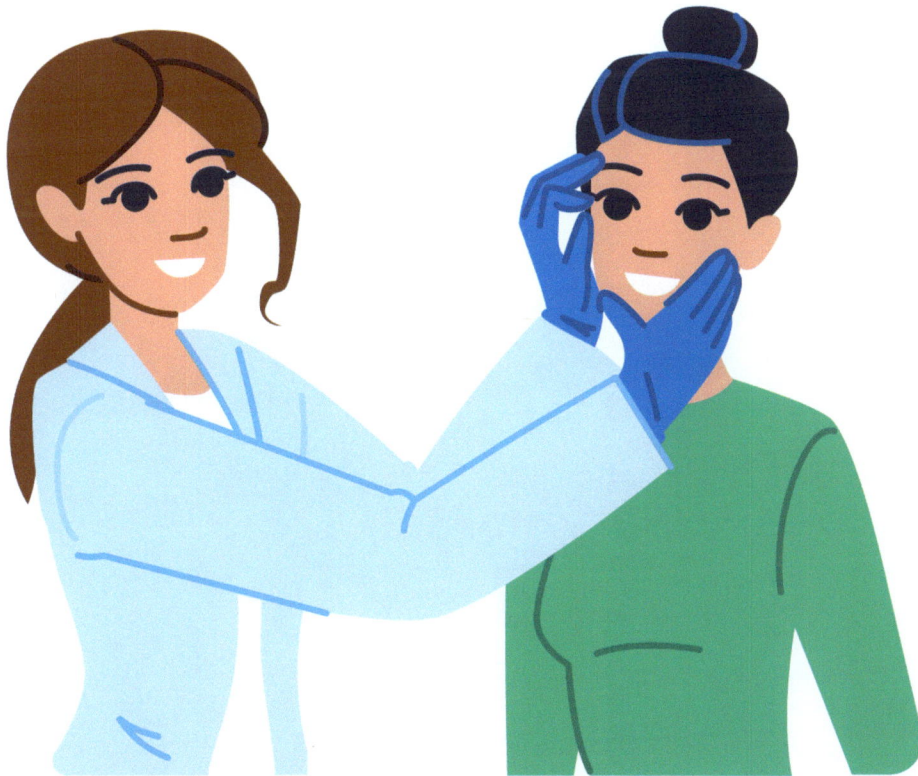

The assessment is entered into the computer.

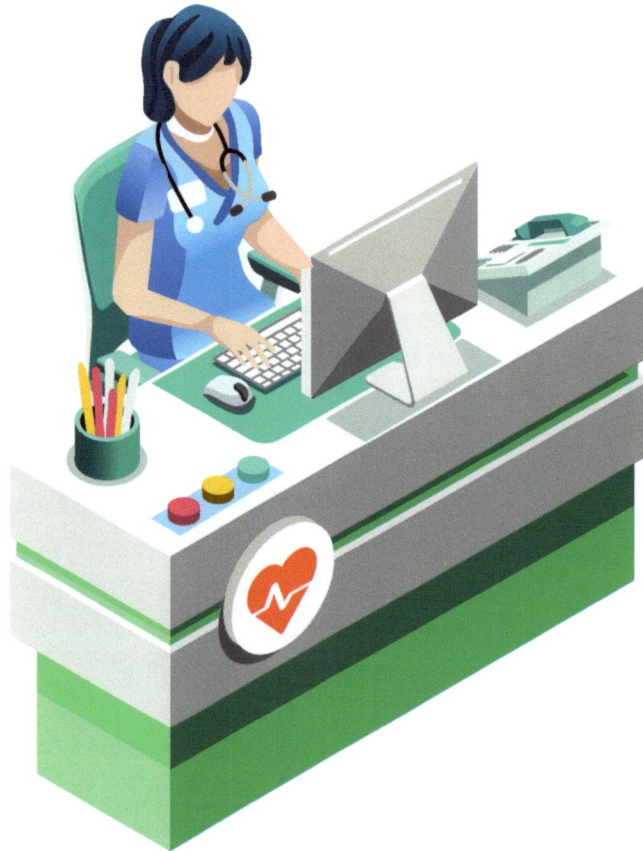

This helps the doctor know whether patients
are getting better or worse.

My Mom talks with so many people at work to make sure that her patients get everything that they need.

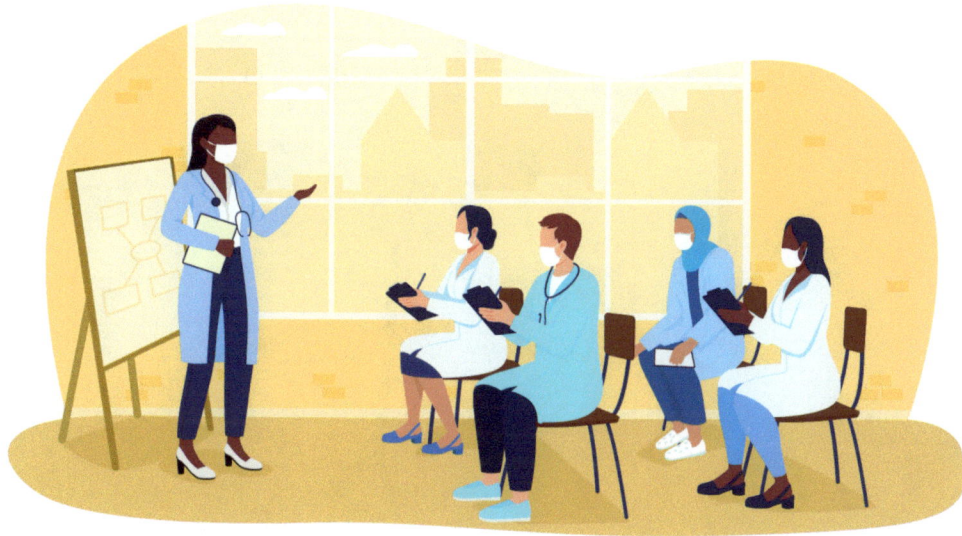

She talks to the doctor to give her report of how her patients are doing.

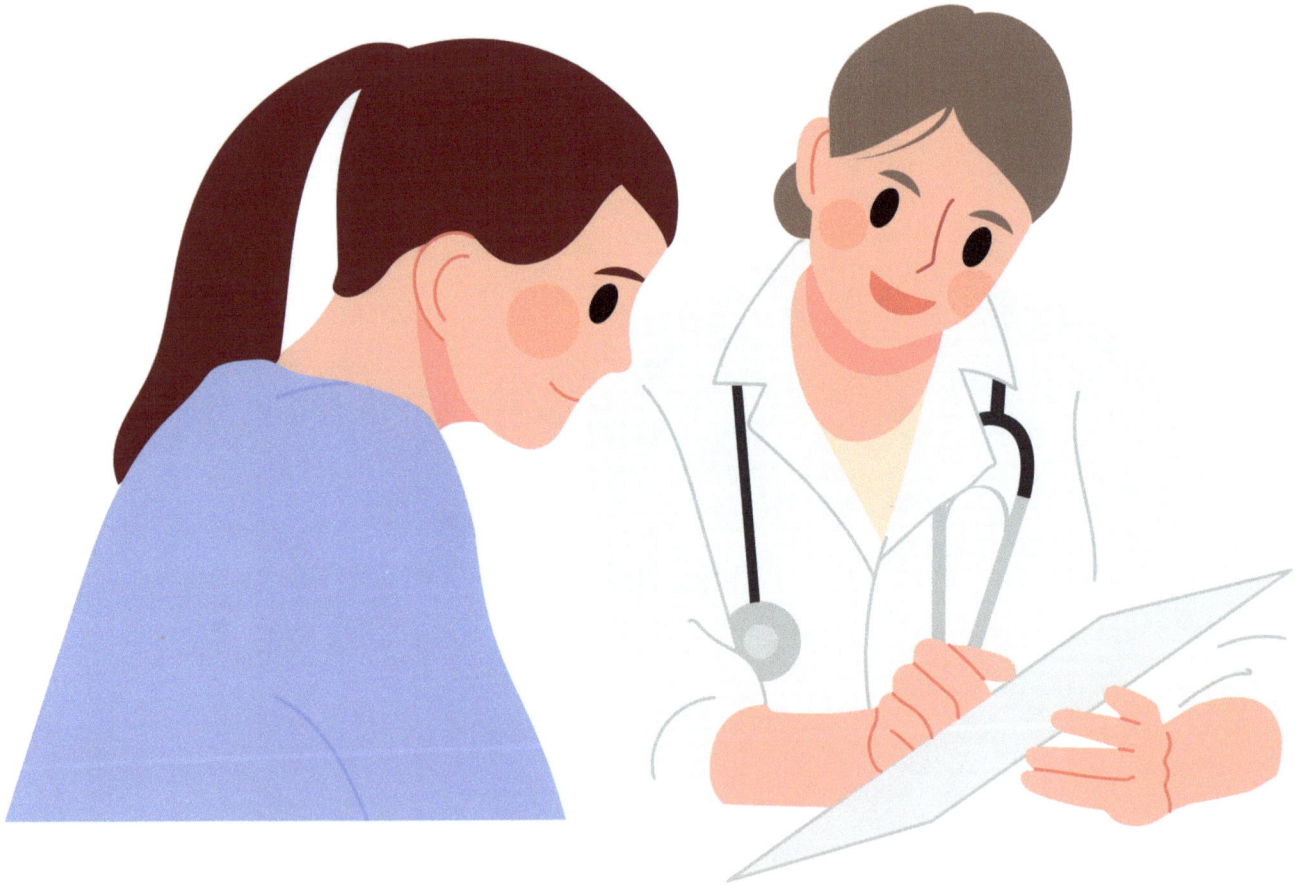

She also gets tasks from doctors when her patients need more assessments, labs, or teaching.

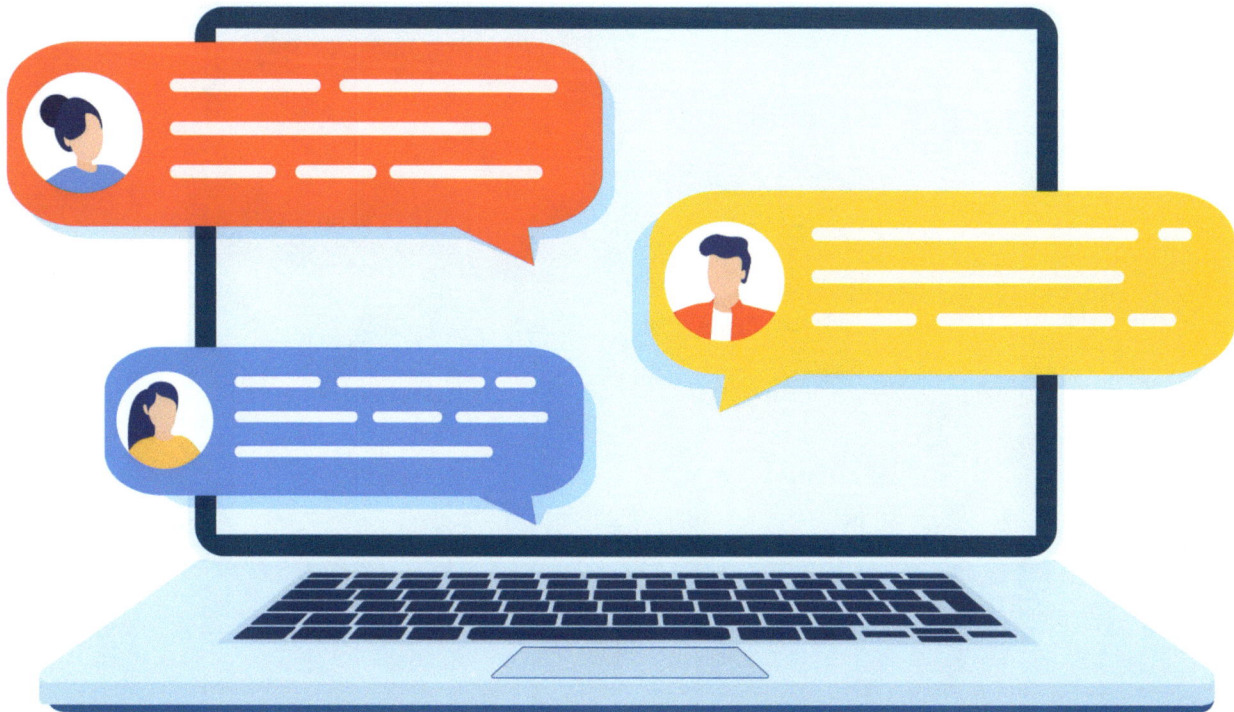

My Mom helps doctors during procedures.

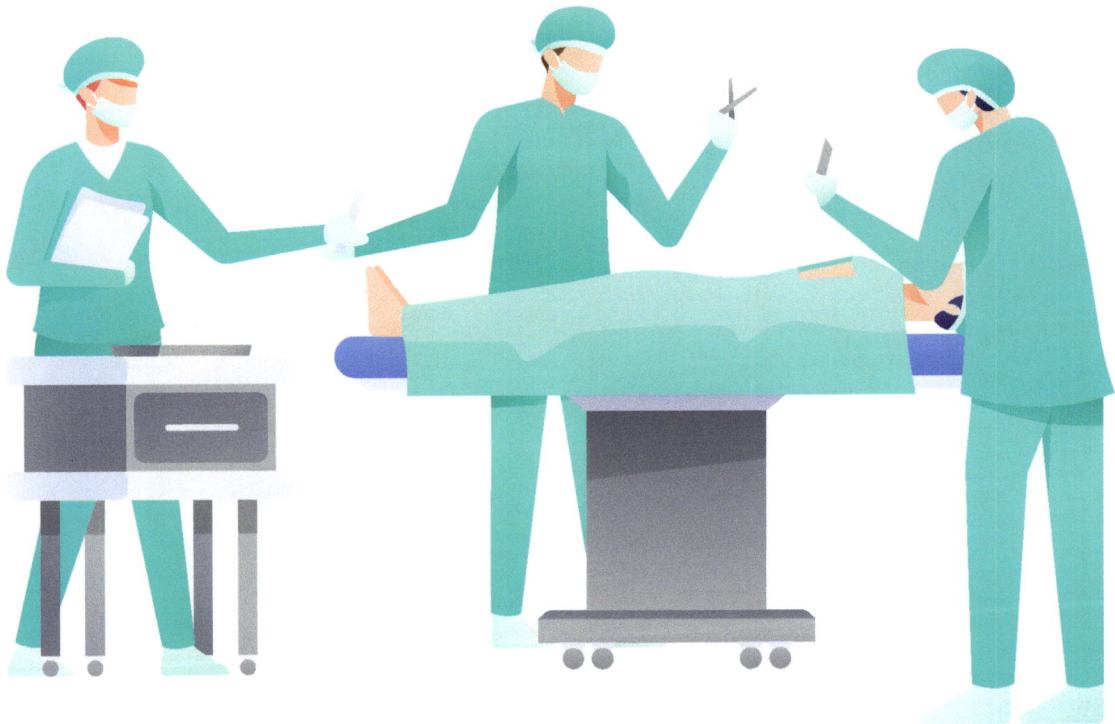

My Mom works with the dietary team to make sure that her patients get their proper meal.

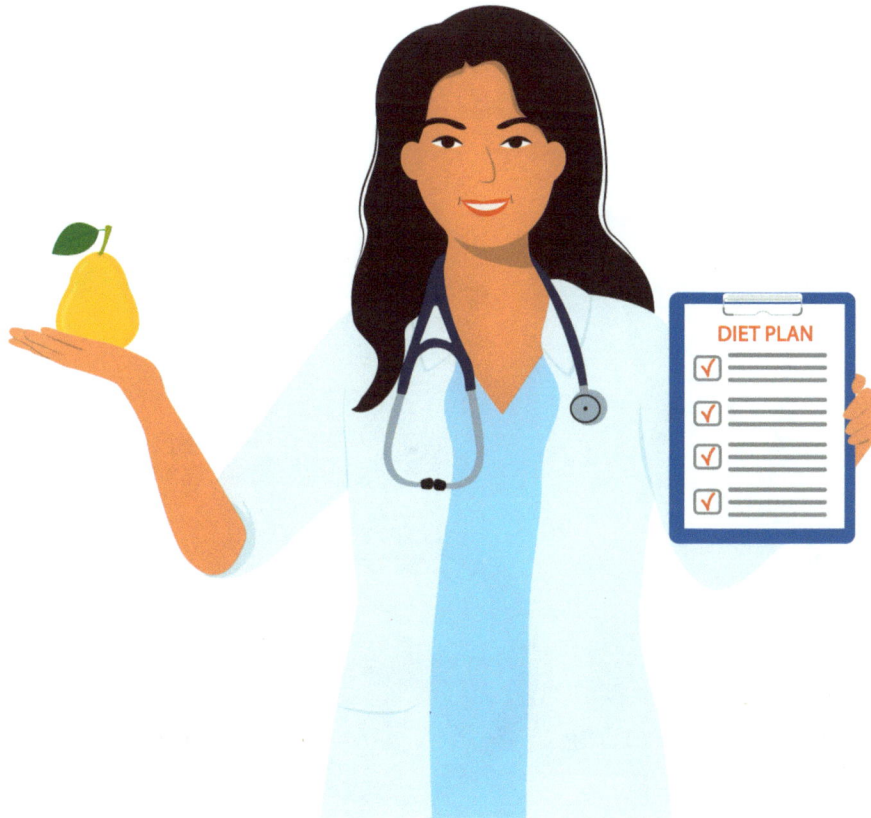

She works with the transportation team when her patients need to go to a test.

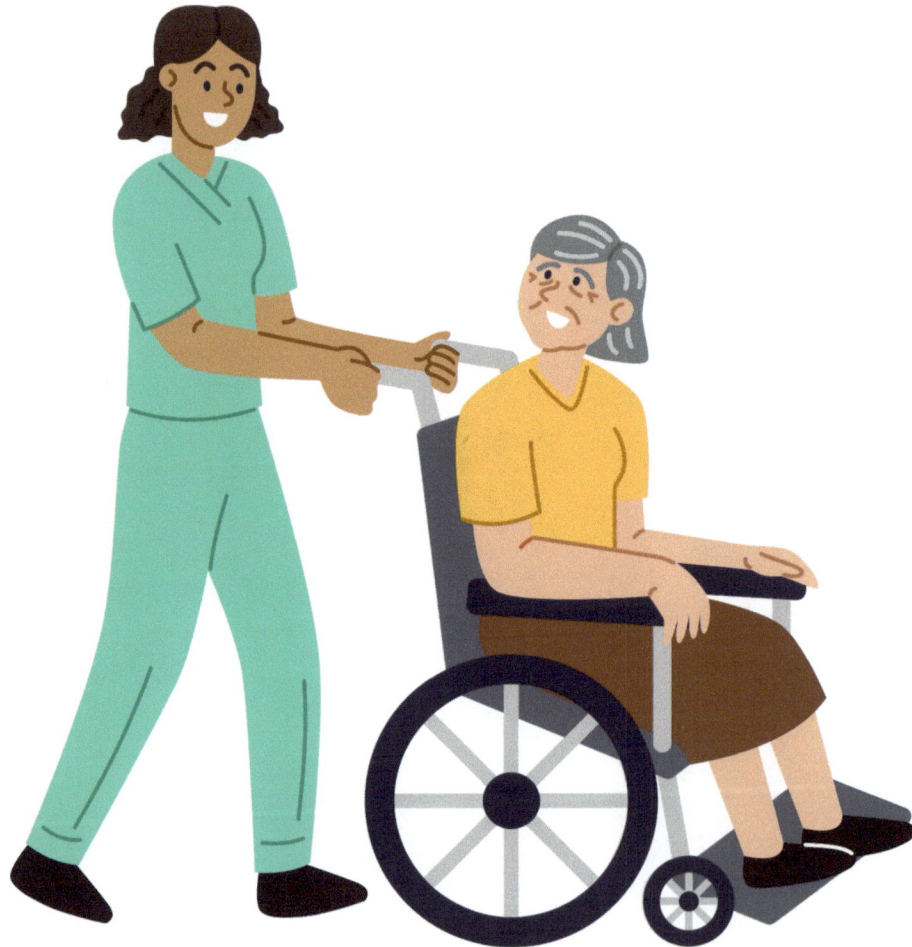

She talks to and helps the physical therapist when they are working with her patient.

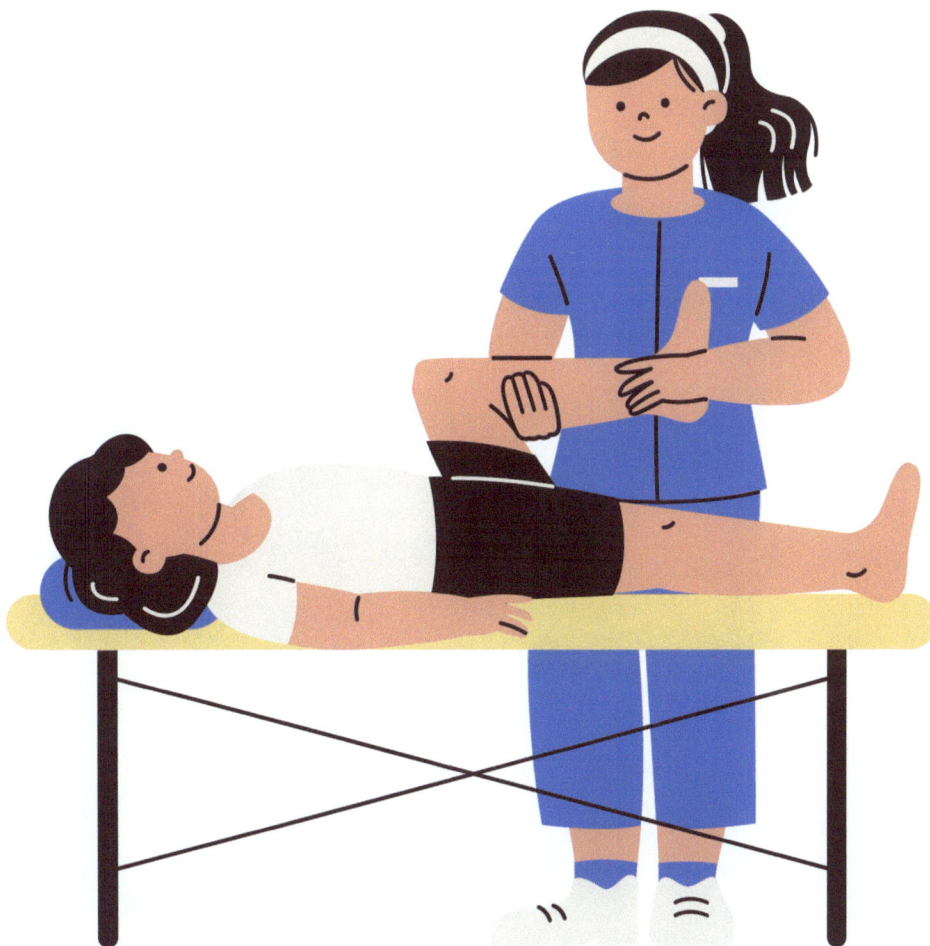

If there is a problem with medications, she talks with a pharmacist.

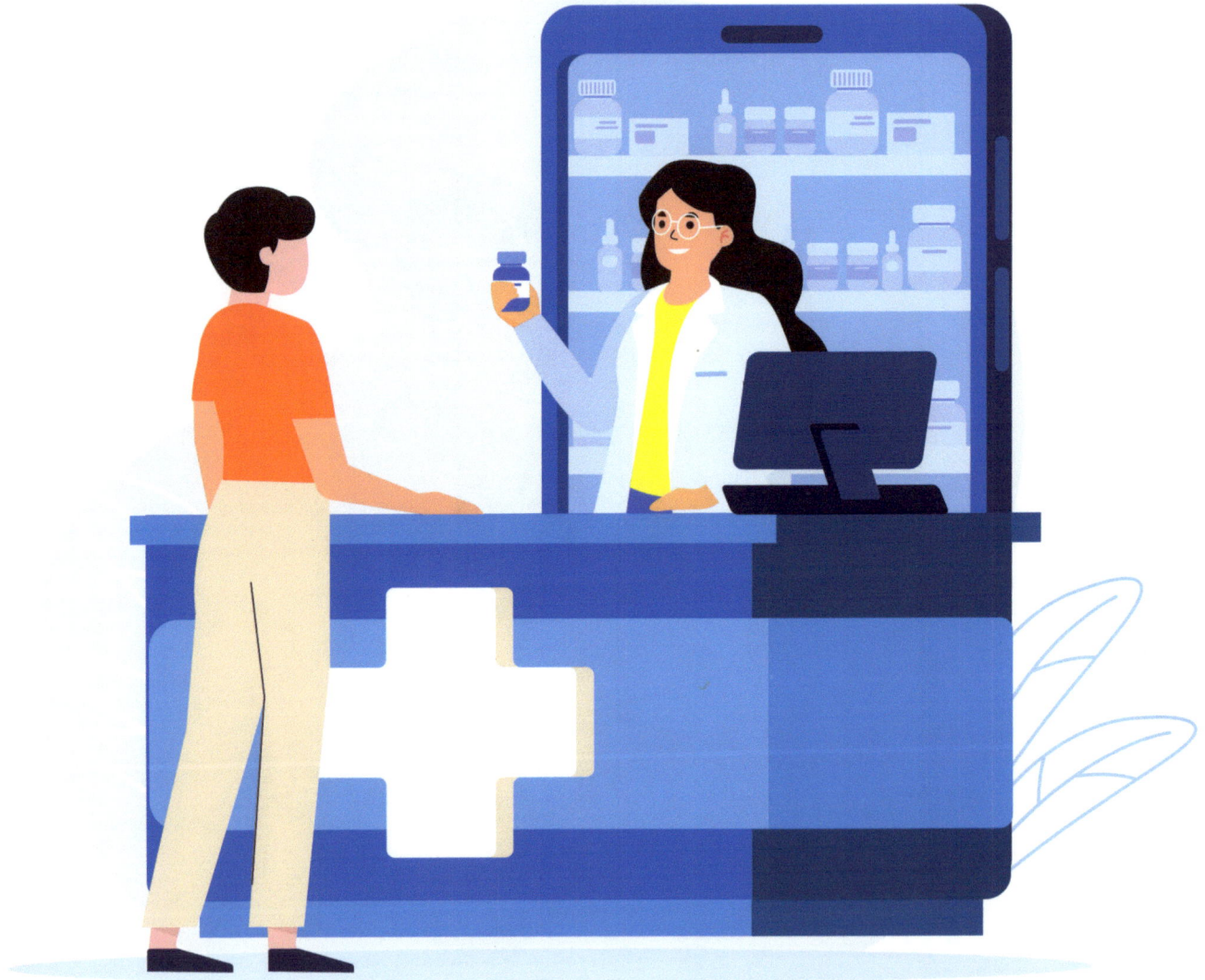

She can even take blood from a patient when the phlebotomist is busy.

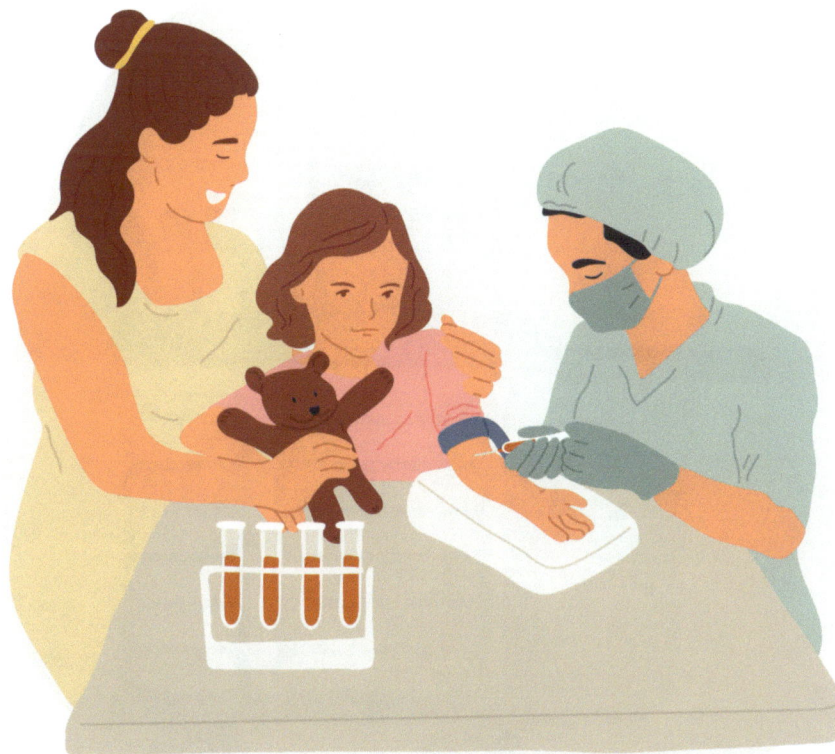

When a patient goes home, she makes sure that the room is ready to be cleaned and calls environmental services.

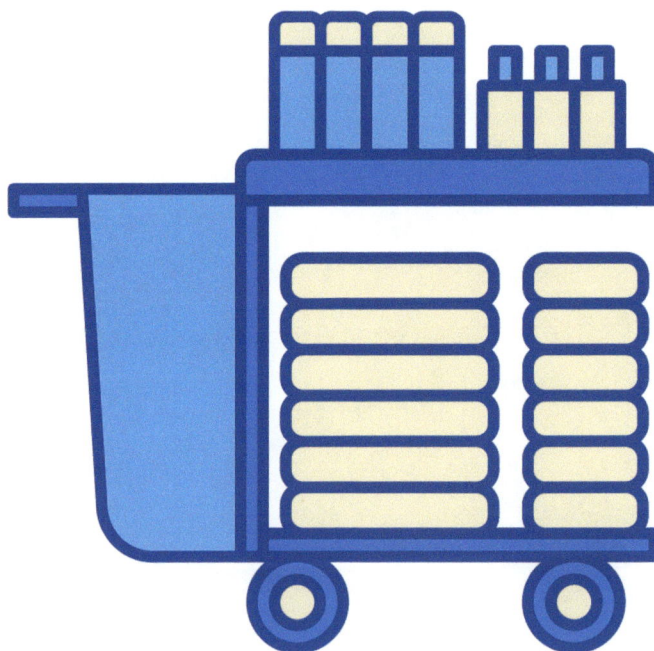

When a family member has a question, they call the nursing station.

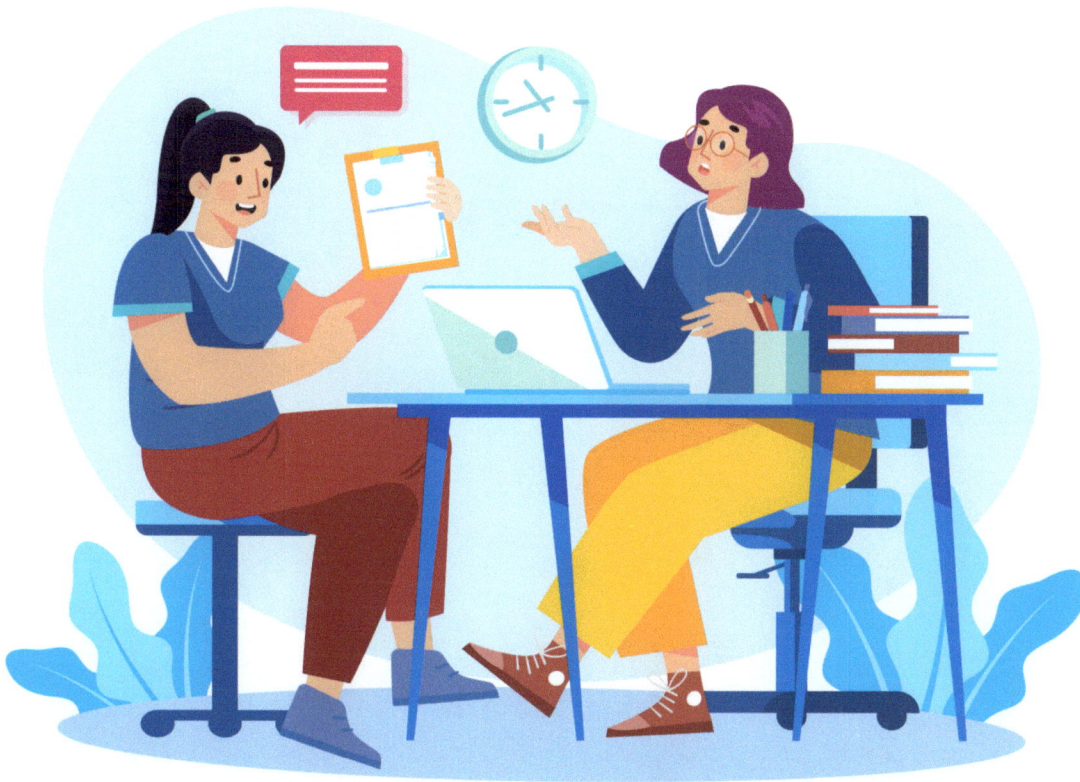

My Mom will either answer the question or help to get the answer.

Sometimes people are not nice to nurses, they yell at them or even try to hit them.

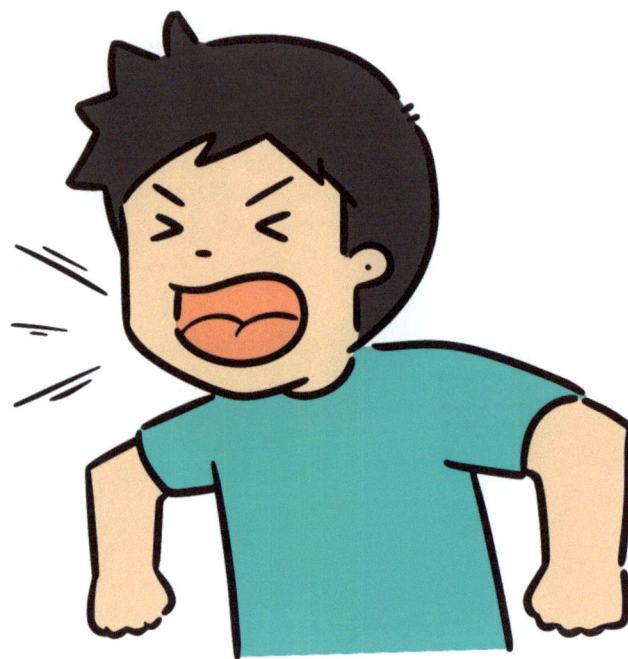

I think that sounds scary.
My Mom says not to worry.

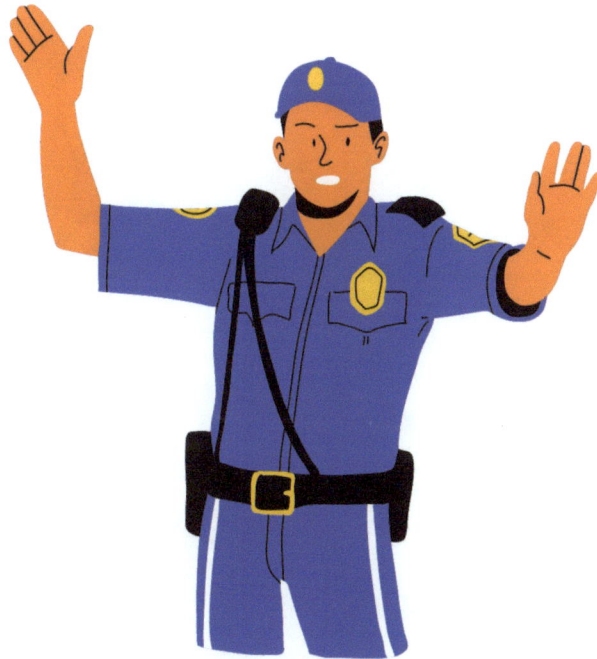

They work together as a team and have the
support of patient safety and security.

Sometimes patients write very nice
thank you notes.

thanks
nurse!

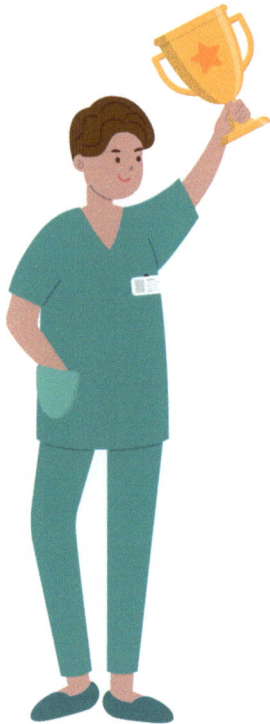

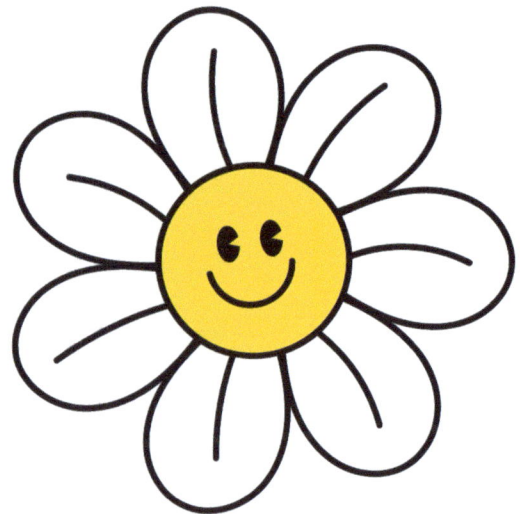

They also nominate my Mom
for special awards.

When I grow up, I want to be a nurse like my Mommy.

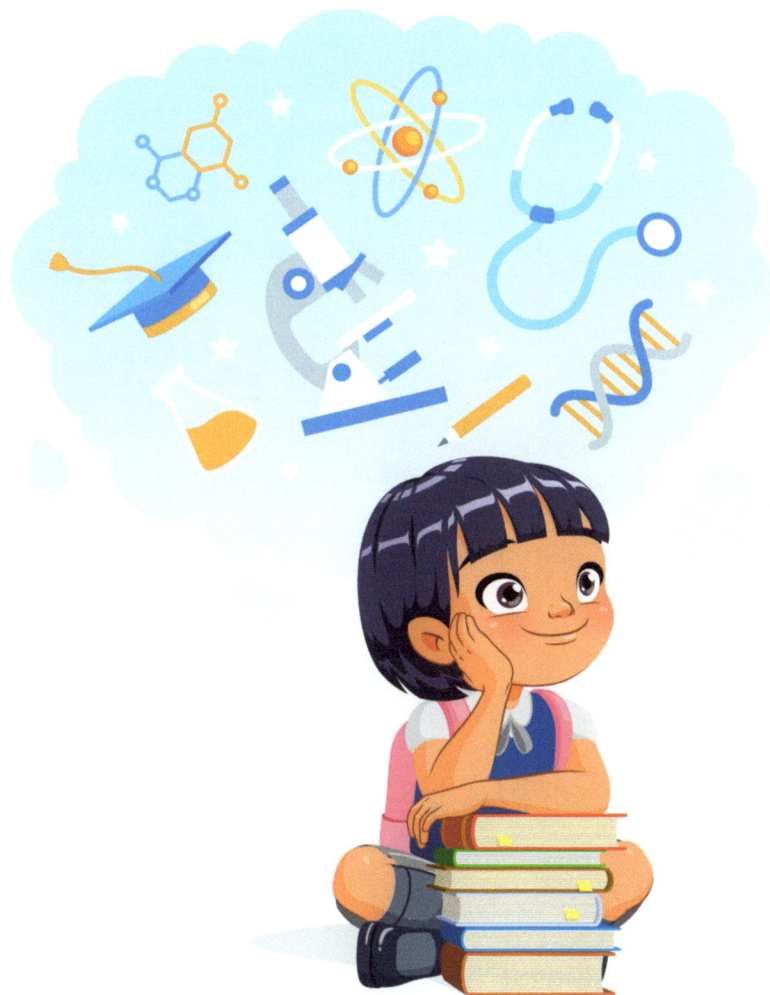

Thank you

If you enjoyed My Mommy Is A Nurse, please check out our other titles and leave a review on Amazon, Goodreads, or your bookstore of choice.

www.ingramcontent.com/pod-product-compliance
Lightning Source LLC
Chambersburg PA
CBHW041105050426
42335CB00046B/141